# Acknowledgements

KT-119-284

I have received invaluable help and support from many people in developing this resource. In particular it would not have been possible without the staff from the seven Teenage Pregnancy Partnerships (TPPs) we have worked with to explore and develop young people's involvement in local strategies. We are extremely grateful to Christine Clark, Cumbria TPP, Kate Jezernik and Frances Newell, Merton TPP, Sue Jablonskas, Nottinghamshire County TPP, Irene Kakoullis, Nottingham City TPP, Julie Husband, Somerset TPP, Sharon Singleton, Suffolk TPP, and Emma Baines and Natalie Wain, Wakefield TPP for the dedication they have shown to the project.

We are also very grateful to members of the project advisory group who guided the Participation in Practice project: Sarah Carter, Regional Teenage Pregnancy Coordinator for the South East, Judith Stonebridge, Sexual Health Manager for Northumberland Teenage Pregnancy Partnership and Judith Green, Sure Start Plus Manager for Nottingham City.

Thanks also to Jo Butcher, Joe Elias and Hanneke Koekkoek at National Children's Bureau for their contributions to the project, and to the Teenage Pregnancy Unit at the Department for Education and Skills for funding the work.

# Foreword by Children's Commissioner for England

I am pleased to introduce this guide. It is a valuable tool for all those working to enable young parents and young people at risk of teenage pregnancy to have a real say in decisions that affect their lives.

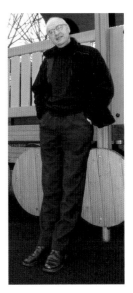

As Children's Commissioner, my role is to promote the views and interests of children and young people in England, especially the disadvantaged and the vulnerable. Teenage parents and young people at risk of teenage pregnancy are a group in particular need of effective support to achieve the five outcomes described in the Green Paper 'Every Child Matters'. Only by actively involving young people in the policies and services developed to meet their needs can we give them the best possible chance of achieving positive outcomes and reduce risks of social exclusion.

Working with young people in a participative way is rewarding for all involved, but involving young people in a meaningful way takes skill, time and commitment. My first year as Commissioner has raised the importance of providing practical tools and support to help practitioners effectively involve young people. I have also been reminded of the need for us all to work in partnership to share ideas and to build new confidence and skills.

The ideas and examples of good practice within this guide demonstrate the excellent work already taking place across the country to involve young people in work to prevent teenage pregnancy and support young parents. I hope that it will inspire colleagues to continue to build new and innovative ways to place the views and experiences of vulnerable young people ever more centrally at the heart of decision-making.

Al Aynsley Green
Children's Commissioner for England

# Foreword by young peer mentor

My name is Chantelle Kay; I am 19 years old and have a beautiful daughter who is nearly two. I work as a peer mentor for Sure Start Plus in Nottingham, helping to make sure that pregnant teenagers and young parents are involved in decisions about their lives and receive the information, advice and support that they need.

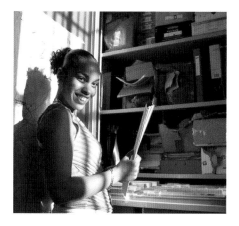

I am a teenage parent myself and feel it is very important that all teenage parents and young people have a voice, a voice to raise their own views and opinions about what they feel is important to them. In order to do this effectively people need to listen to us as we have had real life experiences of being a teenage parent, both negative and positive.

I have been through various different experiences as a teenage parent. I have been in supported accommodation, through the benefits system, in education and also experienced housing problems. I believe that we do not always get to have much involvement in the decisions that are made about our lives, which can make us feel we are being excluded from society. We need to be involved in decisions to make sure that the policies and procedures that are put in place help to meet our needs.

I believe if young people and teenage parents are involved in decision-making it can have a positive effect on society and also the views that teenage parents have towards professionals. It also gives professionals the opportunity to have a better understanding of young people, and their behaviour.

Chantelle Kay
Sure Start Plus peer mentor

# Contents

# 1 Introduction

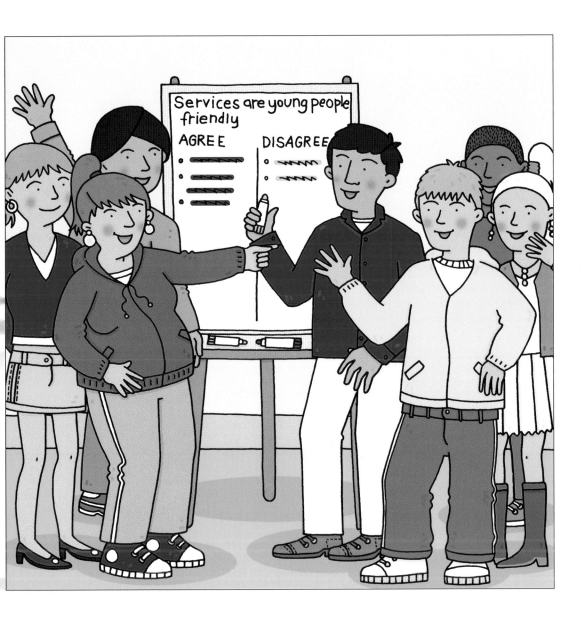

**You need to listen to us to understand what we need!**

**(young person)**

# 1   Introduction

There are endless opportunities for young people to get involved in work to prevent teenage pregnancy, promote sexual health, and support young parents. By creating opportunities for young people to participate in decision-making processes we can make a real difference to their lives, as it helps them to gain confidence and skills to make positive choices about their own health and well-being, and influence how policies and services are developed for young people on a local and national level.

## Background

The National Children's Bureau (NCB) has produced this guide as a result of a two-year national development project funded under the section 64 grant scheme to voluntary organisations administered by the Teenage Pregnancy Unit (TPU) at the Department of Health (from June 2003 at the Department for Education and Skills – DfES). The aim of the project was to improve the quality and quantity of opportunities for young people to participate in local teenage pregnancy strategies. This involved a national mapping exercise to scope the extent and nature of young people's involvement in local strategies. We then invited seven Teenage Pregnancy Partnerships (TPPs) from across the country to work with us to explore and develop young people's involvement in local work in more detail. We worked with the following partnerships:

- Cumbria Teenage Pregnancy Partnership
- Merton Teenage Pregnancy Partnership
- Nottinghamshire County and Nottingham City Teenage Pregnancy Partnerships

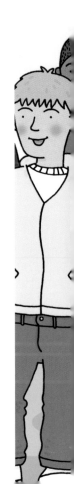

- Somerset Teenage Pregnancy Partnership
- Suffolk Teenage Pregnancy Partnership
- Wakefield Teenage Pregnancy Partnership.

In each area we worked with teenage pregnancy coordinators, youth involvement managers and other key colleagues to review how young people were involved in local strategies and identify priorities for future action. Multi-agency workshops were held at the start of the project to highlight examples of positive practice, discuss challenges for effectively involving young people, and discover opportunities to build on existing work. We then worked alongside our partners to support and encourage young people's participation in decision-making, providing a forum to share good practice and find solutions to common challenges. Throughout the course of the project our partners developed many new and creative opportunities to embed young people's participation into their local strategies. The learning from their experiences forms the basis of this guide.

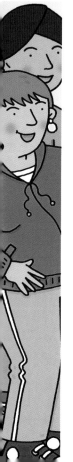

## Who is this guide for?

The guide has been written for all those working to deliver the government's Teenage Pregnancy Strategy. This includes managers and commissioners of services as well as practitioners working with young people across a range of health, youth and community settings. The close links between the Teenage Pregnancy Strategy and wider health, housing and social care provision also makes the guide relevant to all those working to deliver the government's Every Child Matters agenda.

## What does it contain?

The guide contains practical advice and illustrative examples on how to plan, develop and sustain creative opportunities for young people to participate in decision-making.

- *Introduction* provides a background to the guide.

- *Key principles for effective participation* outlines key principles to support practitioners in planning participation work.

- *Participation methods and approaches* provides an outline of different methods and approaches to involve young people in decision-making.

- *Creating the conditions for effective participation* provides a checklist of key principles to help managers build capacity to create participation opportunities for young people.

- *Directory of partners in participation* provides a directory of local partners with a role in creating opportunities for young people to participate in decision-making.

- *References and further information* contains references to sources of useful information.

## Age range

Most of the examples of practice contained within this guide are based on work with young people between the ages of 13 and 19, although the principles apply to work with children and young people of all ages.

## Examples of positive practice

The case studies within this guide will provide ideas and inspiration for developing new ways of involving young people. The examples have been drawn from the TPPs we worked with closely on the project, and from positive work taking place across the country. The criteria for identifying positive practice were that the projects had:

- undertaken a needs assessment

- achieved set objectives

- evaluated outcomes from the work.

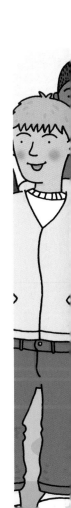

## What do we mean by participation?

Over the past decade there has been growing acceptance of the importance of involving young people in decisions that affect them. The concept of young people's 'participation' has evolved to mean more than young people being present or turning up to a service or event: it is about them being actively involved in making decisions. This includes decisions that are being taken about their own lives, and decisions that affect how policies and services are developed and provided (Willow 2002).

> *It's not just about listening to young people – it's about believing them and acting on what they tell us.*
> *(practitioner)*

Within this guide we use the term 'involvement' interchangeably with the term 'participation' to mean the same thing.

## Why involve young people?

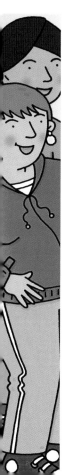

There are many reasons why it is important to involve young people in decisions that affect their lives. Article 12 of the UN Convention on the Rights of the Child (ratified by the UK government in 1991) states that children and young people have a fundamental human right to be involved in decisions that affect their lives. This is increasingly recognised within key government policies affecting children and young people such as the children's National Service Framework (Department of Health 2004a) and the public health White Paper, 'Choosing Health' (Department of Health 2004b). The Children Act (2004) also places great emphasis on the importance of young people's participation. One of the five national outcomes for children and young people outlined in the Every Child Matters programme aims to ensure that all young people have opportunities to 'make a positive contribution' and participate in decisions that affect their lives (Department for Education and Skills 2004).

The Children Act (2004) also created the role of the Children's Commissioner whose function is to promote awareness of views, needs, rights and interests of children and young people, so as to raise their profile and improve their lives and well-being. This includes encouraging people working with children and young people to take account of their views and interests.

## Benefits of involving young people

There are huge benefits to be gained by ensuring that young people are involved in decisions that affect their health and well-being, including the following:

- Young people are empowered to make informed decisions about their own lives.
- Young people have opportunities to have fun and learn new skills that can improve their confidence, health and well-being.
- Young people have the opportunity to influence and improve policies and services for their peers.
- Organisations are more able to provide needs-led services that effectively engage young people because they learn directly about their needs.
- Young people are often really good fun! It can be very enjoyable and fulfilling to work with young people and if you prepare and plan meetings for them, it can make meetings more interesting for all.
- Involving young people can help adults to think more creatively to develop new ideas and solutions.

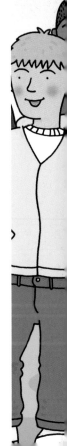

## Who is responsible for young people's participation?

We all have an individual and collective responsibility to reflect on our own work and think about how we might be able to involve young people in the decisions we make. Whatever our role there are opportunities to involve young people. Whether we work directly with young people or are involved in policy and planning, there are many ways in which we can give young people a voice.

The way we involve young people in our work will also depend on the role and function of the organisation we work within. For example, a health clinic that provides direct services to young people will have an important role in ensuring that young people are involved in the design, delivery and evaluation of services. An organisation with a strategic or coordinating role, such as a TPP, might seek to involve young people in specific pieces of work and have an important role in championing and supporting participation among partner agencies.

## Building a culture of participation

For young people to participate in the work of an organisation in a meaningful way, it must be on an ongoing basis rather than via one-off participation activities or events. For this to happen, organisations need to build a culture of participation that encourages and supports young people's involvement in all aspects of its work (Kirby and others 2003).

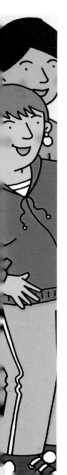

Every organisation is at a different stage in building a culture of participation. Often young people's participation within an organisation starts off at a relatively low level and then grows with time and experience. For example, an organisation might start by consulting young people on decisions made by adults, and then move on to involve young people so they have more power over decisions and help to set the agenda (Hart 1997). Most organisations working with young people strive to involve them at the very highest levels to ensure decisions are firmly rooted in their needs, and to create maximum opportunities for them to develop new skills and confidence.

It can be helpful to think about participation as a journey in which young people's involvement can grow and develop over time (Blake and Frances 2004).

The extent to which young people can influence decisions will depend on many different factors, including time, money, and the amount of commitment there is from those in a position to share power.

## Starting the journey

Those of us who are relatively new to the concept of participation may find the prospect of involving young people in our work slightly daunting at first. A key message from practitioners is that the fear of getting it wrong should not put us off from trying, as we can only develop confidence and learn through experience.

> *You need to be willing to take the risk of involving young people!*
> *(practitioner)*

As you develop more confidence in participation you can increase the opportunities that you offer for young people's involvement.

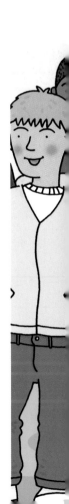

# 2 Key principles for effective participation

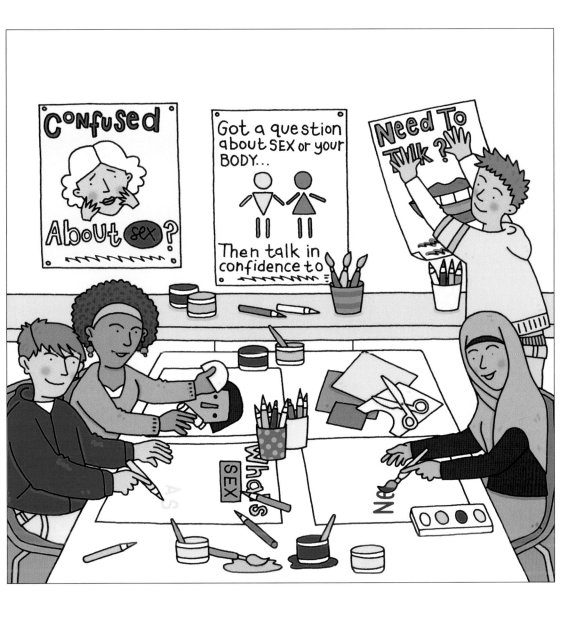

**Our opinions will help you make things better for other young people.**

**(young person)**

# 2 Key principles for effective participation

This section provides an outline and checklist of key principles that we need to consider when planning projects and events to involve young people in decision-making. It also includes practical tips to help ensure that participation work runs smoothly and is as effective as possible.

## Be clear about young people's involvement

It is important to think carefully about exactly what it is that we want young people's views and experiences to influence. We may want their expert insight to inform a specific policy decision we need to make, or to shape the planning or delivery of a service we provide. Whatever the area, it is vital that we set clear parameters for what we hope to achieve so that, in turn, young people feel confident that their involvement is worthwhile and will lead to positive change.

It is important to be open and honest with young people from the start about how much their involvement will influence the final outcome of a decision. It is also important to be clear about the steps that must be taken once their views have been collected so that they understand where the decisions are made and the 'stages of influence'.

## Be flexible

When involving young people in our work we need to be prepared to do things differently. A flexible approach is needed – this might mean

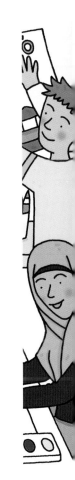

working in the evenings and weekends to fit in with their schedules, changing the format of meetings, and developing different styles of communication.

## Be committed to acting on young people's views

Once we have decided to involve young people in a specific project or initiative it is important that there is consensus among all colleagues involved on the need to act on what we learn from the young people. This also means being prepared to accept criticism.

Unless decision-makers are fully on board it can be very difficult for young people's involvement to have a real impact. If young people do not feel that their efforts have made an impact, they will feel let down and less inclined to take part in future projects.

> *Young people can be cynical that their work won't go anywhere*
> *– it's important that you do what you say you will, and make*
> *sure it happens.*
> *(practitioner)*

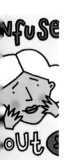

## Make participation enjoyable

To get the most out of young people it is important for participation projects to involve activities that they are likely to enjoy. Drama, dancing, music, film and art can all be a great medium for young people to express their views and opinions. You may want to bring in creative expertise by making links with arts organisations that have experience of working with young people. You can find out about arts organisations in your local area by looking on the Arts Council website at www.artscouncil.org.uk

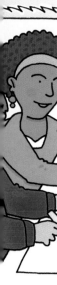

Icebreakers and interactive games can make group work lively and exciting. Organising a hot debate or adapting the format of a popular game show or reality show can also work well to engage young people in discussions. For example, young people might enjoy airing their opinions by talking to Big Brother in a mock diary room, or by thinking about what aspects of a service they would like to put into Room 101 (see Shepherd and Treseder 2002 and McCarthy 2004).

Creative methods are especially effective in engaging more vulnerable young people who may not have the confidence or motivation to get involved with seemingly formal or business-like activities.

Some young people may not feel very excited about participating in a project or event that is explicitly about health issues. Packaging the health focus with a range of activities that young people enjoy is a great way to hook them in and get them interested.

> *If it was just about health then I wouldn't have turned up – it's*
> *good to have lots of different activities.*
> *(young person)*

### Case study: Young dads' viewpoint

Somerset's teenage pregnancy coordinator started a young dads' art project for a number of young fathers across Somerset. This piece of work was part of a South West arts project focusing on young dads. The art project had three main aims: to raise the self-esteem of young fathers, and to counter negative stereotypes of young dads and raise awareness of their needs among the general public.

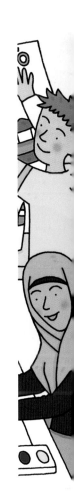

Over the course of six months a participative arts worker worked with individual young dads using photography as a medium for them to explore their experiences of fatherhood. The young dads were taught some basic photographic techniques and were lent digital cameras to capture images of their lives and their relationships with their children. They also had their photograph taken with their children and were each given a framed picture to keep. The work was then put together in a published booklet to highlight their thoughts, feelings and experiences on what it means to be a young father. The booklet has been widely disseminated – the photographs were part of an art exhibition in Bristol and framed copies of them are on display at local maternity units.

The photographs have also been made into an interactive DVD where viewers can click on the photographs to hear the young fathers talking about their needs and experiences. Professionals were able to view the DVD at a county conference that highlighted the needs of young parents. Local area events and networks have been set up to take action on points raised at the conference. The issues raised by the young fathers have also been incorporated into a young parents' guide called TiPs, which is distributed by Connexions.

The young fathers enjoyed participating in the project and, for some, it has been a stepping-stone for their participation in further work.

**Key learning**: The young men were clearly very proud of their achievements, and this highlighted the importance of ensuring that they gained appropriate rewards and recognition for their work. This was achieved by giving each young dad a large wooden-framed copy of his photograph in addition to the usual thank-you letters.

**Contact**: Julie Husband, Somerset Teenage Pregnancy Partnership
Jhusband@connexions-somerset.org.uk
01823 320 309

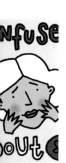

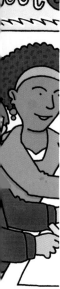

## Ensure broad representation

To ensure that participation work reflects the diverse needs of young people it is important that a representative group is involved. We need to consider which groups of young people will be affected by the decisions we are making and how we can target a cross-section in terms of their age, gender, ethnicity and background.

Working in partnership with other agencies can be a good way of ensuring that our work includes a broad cross-section of young people with different needs. For example, we can access vulnerable groups by making links with local substance-misuse services, youth homelessness projects or Youth Offending Teams.

To make sure that work is inclusive of young people from minority ethnic backgrounds make links with local community or faith groups. If young people from minority ethnic groups are under-represented in local services, you could develop a project to uncover their views on how services could be developed to meet their needs.

It is also important to ensure that disabled young people are supported so that they can inform decision-making processes. There are a number of guides containing further information on the practicalities of ensuring that participation work is inclusive of disabled young people (see Morris 1998 and Kirkbride 1999).

### Case study: Bollywood health event

Nottingham City Teenage Pregnancy Partnership organised a targeted health event to ensure that the local teenage pregnancy strategy addressed the needs of young people from Asian communities. The aim of the event was to enable young people to have fun while also consulting them about their health needs and providing information and advice in a non-threatening way.

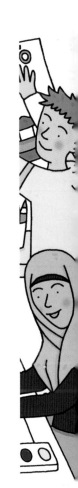

Asian young people were asked what sort of event they would like and they suggested a Bollywood theme would be a good idea. The event took place at a cinema so that young people could watch a film and then wander round various stands offering health needs assessments, information and treats including massage and henna tattoos. The local chlamydia screening service was present on the day and reported that Asian young women visited the service following the event.

Findings from the health needs assessments have been used in the local Children and Young People's Plan, and particular issues have been included in the development of a local standard for 'young-people-friendly services'.

Following feedback from young people at the event, a further health event was planned for Asian young men who stated that they wanted to have the opportunity to explore sexual health issues in single-sex groups. An MOT (Men-Only Time) event was held for Asian young men during the summer of 2005.

**Key learning**: The success of the event emphasises the importance of offering young people fun activities as an incentive to engage in health education and promotion initiatives.

**Contact**: Irene Kakoullis, Nottingham City Teenage Pregnancy Partnership
Irene.Kakoullis@nottinghamcity.gov.uk
0115 915 7028

## Consider young people's access needs

It is important to organise participation activities so that they fit in around young people and do not interrupt their commitments to education or employment – this can mean organising meetings and events in the evening or at weekends. A suitable venue is also important. This should be conveniently located, accessible for young people who may have a disability, and be the kind of space where young people can feel relaxed and safe.

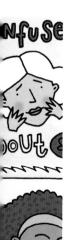

### A lesson learned...

*When planning an event for homeless young people we thought it would be a bit of a treat for them to go to a nice hotel, but when we got there the formal atmosphere made the young people feel uncomfortable and a few of them thought that the staff were looking down on them. When it came to lunch time some of the young people felt intimidated by the formality of the dining room and chose to go outside for fast food instead. The experience enabled me to realise the importance of choosing a venue for participation events where young people are likely to feel respected and at ease.*
*(practitioner)*

How young people will get to the venue is another factor to consider. They may be able to get a lift with a parent or carer, or it might be necessary to arrange taxis or a minibus. If young people are travelling on public transport then it is good practice to make sure that their travel costs are either paid in advance or reimbursed.

## Create a safe and healthy environment

When planning participation projects it is crucial to ensure that there will be enough suitably experienced staff to supervise the work. All staff working with children and young people will need to have an understanding of basic child protection and be checked by the Criminal Records Bureau. When working with young people aged under 18, it may be necessary to get parental consent for them to take part in certain activities, especially if they are being filmed or photographed.

As well as providing a little incentive for young people to attend meetings or events, drinks and snacks are important for keeping young people's concentration and energy levels up. Check for specialist dietary requirements in advance. Offering healthy choices such as fruit juices, sandwiches and cereal bars is a good way to promote healthy lifestyles.

## Provide incentives for young people

The decision on whether or not it is appropriate to pay young people for their involvement in our work will depend on a number of factors, including their age and occupational status, and what is being asked of them in terms of the time and effort they will have to dedicate. If young people are expected to give up a lot of time and provide a service (such as peer research or facilitation) then it seems fair that they are paid.

You may want to reward young people for their contributions in other ways, such as by giving them gift vouchers or organising a day trip or fun activity. If you are planning to involve young people in a project that offers significant learning and development opportunities, it is worth considering whether there is scope to gain formal accreditation from a local college or a recognised national body (for example, see the National Open College Network, www.nocn.org.uk, or ASDAN, www.asdan.org.uk).

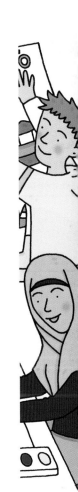

**A lesson learned...**

*I once organised an event to consult young people on a new government policy. I had enough money in the budget to give young people a £10 voucher for their time and thought it would be a good incentive to get them along. Although lots of young people did turn up, I soon realised that I hadn't given enough thought to the format of the session. The young people soon got bored of answering my questions and the discussion lost momentum. Some of the young people admitted that they were only there to get the voucher and weren't really interested in taking part in the discussions. The experience taught me to think more creatively about how to encourage young people to participate in future work, and not to rely on vouchers as a way to capture their interest. It also taught me to plan the format of similar events so that it is fun and engaging and offers an incentive within itself for young people to want to get involved. (practitioner)*

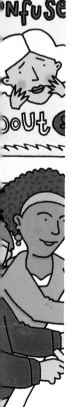

## Provide young people with feedback

It is important that we show young people how their views have influenced decision-making processes and affected outcomes. There are many different ways of providing this crucial feedback, such as giving young people reports or arranging face-to-face meetings with key stakeholders. It is important to think of a way of providing feedback that is enjoyable for young people. You may want to organise an event with a dual purpose of feeding information back to young people and celebrating their valued contributions.

## Celebrate young people's achievements

There are many ways we can help celebrate what young people achieve through their participation in projects and events. As well as thank-you letters, giving awards and certificates can be a way of showing young people that their contributions are valued. Organising special events or outings can also be a great way to celebrate and reward young people for their involvement in your work.

### Case study: Film gets premiere event

Nottinghamshire County Teenage Pregnancy Partnership worked with 36 young people to develop a film, *Making your mind up*, on the subject of sex and relationships. The film has been produced as a resource to support the delivery of sex and relationships education. Open auditions were held to recruit young people to take part in the film, and those chosen for parts were consulted on the scripts.

The young people involved in the project were enthusiastic and recognised that their participation in the project would make an important difference to the education of their peers. The young people acknowledged that as a result of their involvement in the project they had gained confidence and a greater understanding of sex and relationships issues.

> *I have gained a lot of knowledge...it has given me a lot of confidence.*
> *(young person)*

A premiere event was organised at a local cinema to launch the film and celebrate young people's contributions to the project. The local press were there to take photos of the young people as they arrived. The cinema was decorated with flowers, balloons and posters of the film, and canapés and fruit punch were on tap, prepared and served by catering students from a local college. After the film was shown, two locally born TV actors congratulated the young people and presented them with certificates and copies of the film.

**Key learning**: The success of the event and the positive feedback from young people served as a reminder of the importance of demonstrating to young people that their contributions are valued.

**Contact**: Sue Jablonskas, Nottinghamshire Teenage County Pregnancy Partnership
Sue.Jablonskas@nottscc.gov.uk
01623 627 322

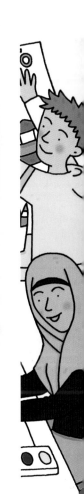

## Evaluate and build on young people's involvement

Once a participation project or event has finished, it is important to reflect on what worked well and what could have been improved – this will inform how we do things in the future. We need to keep building on our experiences to develop new and creative ways for young people to get involved.

Also, it is also important to keep building on the work because young people who have had a positive experience of participating are likely to be keen to remain involved in future work to take forward the ideas and recommendations that emerge.

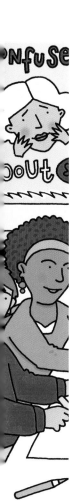

---

### Checklist of key principles for young people's participation

Is there a clear purpose to young people's involvement? ❑

Are you prepared to do things differently? ❑

Is there is a commitment to act on young people's views? ❑

Have you decided how to make the work fun and creative? ❑

Have you considered how the work will be representative? ❑

Have you considered young people's access needs? ❑

Have you considered how to create a safe and positive environment? ❑

Have you decided what payments or incentives to offer young people? ❑

Have you considered how you will provide young people with feedback? ❑

Have you considered how you plan to celebrate young people's achievements? ❑

Is there a commitment to evaluate and build on young people's involvement? ❑

# 3 Participation methods and approaches

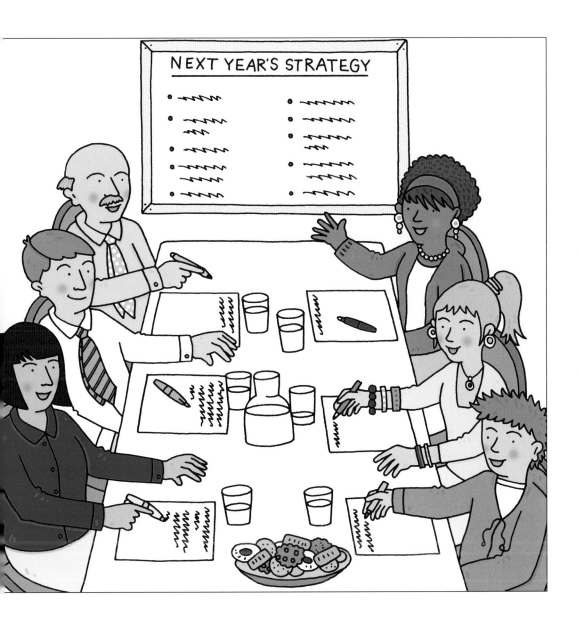

**It's important to see things from our point of view.**

**(young person)**

# 3 Participation methods and approaches

This section provides an overview of some of the main approaches used to involve young people in decision-making processes.

The most appropriate method will depend on a number of factors, including the type of decision you want young people to influence, the age and maturity of the young people you are working with, and the amount of time and resources available to dedicate to their involvement. Most methods can be applied and adapted to suit a range of different contexts.

## Helping young people to make informed decisions

For those of us providing direct services to young people, a key focus of our day-to-day work is on supporting their full involvement in the decisions they make about their own lives. In order to make informed decisions, young people need support to recognise and fully understand their options.

### Active listening

It is often the time we spend informally listening to young people and answering their questions that makes the real difference in terms of their ability to make informed decisions. An atmosphere where young people feel confident to seek support, ask questions, and talk openly about their health and well-being needs is crucial. This requires us to develop effective skills in communicating with young people (see Jones 2003 or Brody 1998).

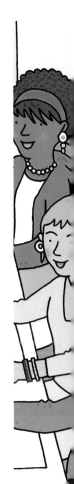

There are a number of ways in which services can maximise opportunities for adults to spend time listening to young people – for example, some health services have increased time slots for check-ups with young people, to build up that all-important rapport and allow extra time for questions.

## Accessible information and advice

Young people need access to written information in a format that is clear and easy for them to understand. One of the best ways to make sure that information contained in leaflets, websites and other resources is appropriate to young people's needs is to involve them in writing and developing them!

## Peer support

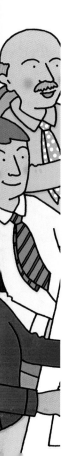

Peer support schemes can be an excellent way to increase young people's ability to make informed decisions. Young people who have had a common experience can be in a good position to guide others and provide support in a style that responds to their needs. In addition to listening to young people, peer support workers can also help to signpost young people to relevant services and advocate on their behalf. There are many different settings in which peer support schemes can be developed, including schools, prisons, housing, and health services (see Hartley-Brewer 2002 or McGowan 2002).

### Case study: Peer antenatal support group

Cumbria Teenage Pregnancy Partnership worked with a young parent to pilot a peer antenatal support group for expectant teenage parents. The group was formed in response to evidence that some young people were not accessing existing antenatal services as they found them intimidating and adult-focused.

At the outset of the project the young parent consulted her peers on the issues they wanted the group to cover. She found that alongside conventional antenatal advice they wanted support on a wider variety of issues, including advice on their entitlement to housing and benefits, education and training, and support to develop life-skills such as cooking. She then developed a 10-week course to address these issues, which ran three times with different groups of expectant parents over the course of the pilot.

Outcomes from the pilot have been very positive. The antenatal support group has now been mainstreamed within local health services and is coordinated by a dedicated teenage pregnancy liaison midwife. Young people work in partnership with the midwife to ensure that the service develops around their needs. They have been involved in organising 'outward bound' trips and now want to gain formal accreditation for the learning opportunities provided within the group. The young parent who piloted the group also gained valuable skills from her involvement in the project and has moved on to study for a degree in youth and community studies.

**Key learning**: Holding the group sessions in a community setting rather than a clinical setting helped to create a more relaxed and informal atmosphere.

**Contact**: Christine Clark, Cumbria Teenage Pregnancy Partnership
Christine.clark@cumbriacc.gov.uk
01228 601 207

## Involving young people in the design and delivery of services

It is important that we capture young people's experiences to learn how we can further improve the support provided to meet their needs. There are many ways in which we can involve young people in the design and delivery of services.

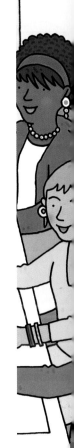

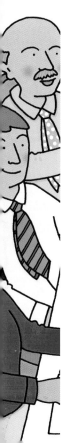

## Informal evaluation by local practitioners

Those working with young people on a day-to-day basis often gain a unique insight into young people's lives in relation to their experiences of services and the policies we develop to meet their needs. It is important that this knowledge and expertise is harnessed to complement formal methods of evaluating young people's experiences.

Although this is likely to happen on an informal basis, some organisations have introduced formal systems to make sure that this knowledge is not lost. For example, some teenage pregnancy coordinators set aside time during meetings with local practitioners for focused discussion on key issues and concerns raised by young people.

## Service user surveys

Surveys can be a simple and useful way of gathering the views of large numbers of young people on the accessibility and quality of services. There are ways that this process can be developed to increase young people's participation – such as involving young people in the design of forms and challenging them to think of ways the format can be made fun and engaging.

## Service user groups

Many services set up regular meetings as a forum to consult people on their experiences of using services and to inform future plans. Services that work with all age groups will need to think about how young people are encouraged to take part in this type of meeting. Young people might feel intimidated or out of place in meetings they perceive to be adult-focused, so it is important to think of ways to create a relaxed and informal atmosphere.

## Mystery shoppers

'Mystery shopper' schemes are a really good way of involving young people in the evaluation of services. They usually consist of a group of young people 'going undercover' to judge the extent to which the service they received was 'young-people-friendly' and make recommendations on how aspects of the service could be improved. This method works well in various settings, including GP surgeries, sexual health clinics, advice centres and pharmacies.

**Case study: Undercover – young people evaluate sexual health services**

As part of Sheffield's teenage pregnancy strategy, young people have been involved in the evaluation of clinic-based and outreach sexual health services using a 'mystery shopper' approach (i.e. young people presenting themselves as an ordinary service user). The aim of the work is to ensure that services are accessible and appropriate for young people, and enable them to have an active voice in the quality and type of services provided.

The teenage pregnancy youth participation worker at the Centre for HIV and Sexual Health recruited a group of 10 young people from local schools, colleges and voluntary projects to take part in the project. They received training that outlined their roles and responsibilities and set parameters for the aspects of services to be evaluated – such as their accessibility and the quality of the physical environment. The training also covered confidentiality issues and an outline of the limits of the evaluation, such as not allowing any tests or physical examinations to be carried out on them.

An evaluation checklist was prepared in discussion with the nine services that volunteered to take part in the project. Following the visits young people made a number of recommendations on how aspects of the services could be improved, such as the need for more youth-friendly reading materials in waiting areas, and better soundproofed rooms for confidential discussion. They also recommended that services should be

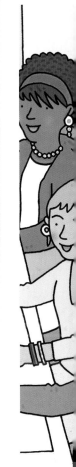

more clearly signposted and suggested that publicity leaflets should include a mini street map and information about bus routes.

Young people were also involved in feedback meetings with each service to discuss how suggested recommendations were to be implemented. Young people participating in the project have reported feeling increasingly confident and many have gone on to participate in other initiatives, such as the production of a video, *Undercover Uncovered*, which outlines the process of involving young people in undercover evaluations.

**Key learning**: Outcomes from the scheme highlight the importance of working closely with services to help prepare them for the evaluation, because otherwise, some services might find it difficult to embrace young people's views and recommendations. Other key learning includes the importance of allowing sufficient time between the initial and follow-up visits to enable staff to implement changes.

**Contact**: Liz Murray, Centre for HIV and Sexual Health
Liz.Murray@chiv.nhs.uk
0114 226 1915

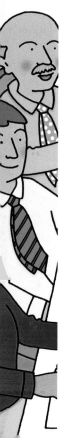

### Case study: Helping GPs to be youth-friendly

Young people in Stoke have been involved in an exciting project to help general practitioners (GPs) make their sexual health services attractive and accessible for young people.

The first stage of the work involved a group of young people undertaking random checks of GP surgeries to observe how 'young-people-friendly' they were. The young people reported that there was lots of scope for improvement and recommended that a scheme was needed to support GPs make improvements to their surgeries. The Developing Adolescent Sexual Health (DASH) project was then set up to help GPs implement the toolkit, *Getting it Right for Teenagers in Your Practice*, which offers practical suggestions on how GP surgeries can be made more attractive and accessible to young people. The toolkit, produced in 2002 by the Royal College of Nursing and the Royal College of General Practitioners, aims to help GPs make sure that their practices are 'teenager-friendly'. Ten GP surgeries across North Staffordshire are working as DASH pilots to introduce a range of improvements, such as sending birthday cards to invite young people for health checks, training for staff in effectively communicating with young people, and putting up dedicated notice boards for young people in waiting rooms. Once the services have had time to implement improvements the young people will be conducting a 'mystery shopper' exercise to review how services have improved.

Young people have also been involved in developing a 'rough guide' to accessing GP surgeries to highlight the fact that the services offered by GPs are confidential. A project to involve young people in an audit of the provision of emergency contraception by pharmacy services is also under way.

**Key learning**: The work highlights the importance of providing partners with an incentive to hook them into projects to improve services. Providing tools, support and encouragement is vital to ensuring that recommendations are taken forward and implemented.

**Contact**: Jane Mayer, North Staffordshire NHS Trust
Jane.Mayer@northstaffs.nhs.uk
01782 425 931

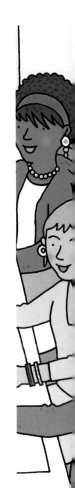

## Participation and consultation events

Consultation events are a useful way to help build understanding of an issue and identify opportunities for further work. For example, an organisation may want to consult young people on a plan or policy they are developing, or on their experiences of a service to inform decisions about future service design and delivery (see Fajerman and others 2000).

**Case study: Drama gets young fathers involved**

Merton Teenage Pregnancy Partnership developed a unique project to increase involvement of young fathers in their local strategy and inform future provision to meet their needs. The views and experiences of young fathers were canvassed via group and individual interviews. The findings were then turned into a short play by a theatre company and performed at a consultation event attended by 30 young fathers. The play was successful at prompting discussion about how local services could be improved and a number of recommendations emerged from the event – including the need for better access to housing advice and opportunities to develop parenting skills.

The project helped to provide a sound evidence base to expand support available to young fathers in Merton. Since the event a number of the young fathers have made use of teenage parent support services and engaged positively in other projects and initiatives. The event was successful on a number of levels as it helped professionals to increase their understanding of the needs of young fathers, while also raising awareness among young fathers about the services and support already available.

**Key learning**: Using drama helped to create a safe space for young people to discuss their views, as they were able to relate their own experiences to those of the characters and reveal as little or as much personal information as they felt comfortable with.

**Contact**: Kate Jezernik, Merton Teenage Pregnancy Partnership
Kate.Jezernik@smpctnurses.nhs.uk
020 8687 4733

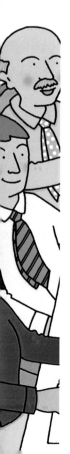

Peer research

There are many positive benefits to be gained from involving young people in the design and delivery of research projects. Young researchers are in a position to gather rich insights, as their peers may feel more relaxed and open talking to them about health and well-being issues than they might when talking to adult researchers. This method also creates opportunities for the young people carrying out the research to gain new skills such as developing research questions, interview techniques, and analysing and presenting findings (see Kirby 1999 and Worall 2000).

### Case study: South Asian young people investigate sex and relationships

Blackburn with Darwen Teenage Pregnancy Partnership worked with the Centre of Ethnicity and Health at the University of Central Lancashire (UCLAN) to involve young people of South Asian heritage in an innovative peer research project.

The aim of the research project was to gain a better understanding of the sexual health needs of young people of South Asian heritage to inform future service developments. It was initiated in response to evidence that young women of South Asian heritage accounted for 1 in 8 of all requests for terminations, yet made up only 1 in 20 of those accessing general sexual health information or contraception.

Ten young people of South Asian heritage were recruited to take part in the project. They were all paid £5 per hour for the time they gave to it. The young people were trained in research skills by UCLAN, including questionnaire design, interview methods and data analysis techniques. They targeted their peers in various venues to complete the questionnaire and run focus groups. They also organised a Bangra event as a fun way to engage other young people in the project.

Findings from the work revealed that almost half of the young people had not received any sexual health education, and that concerns about confidentiality were often a major barrier to accessing local services. They also highlighted the fact that strong family, religious and cultural influences may affect young people's decisions about whether or not to use contraception, both inside and outside of marriage. Recommendations from the project have been incorporated into the local strategy. This has led to action to produce targeted information campaigns for young people of South Asian heritage, and work with local services to improve the development and promotion of confidentiality policies.

**Key learning**: It was initially planned that the young researchers would organise a number of focus groups with their peers. However, several of the young people were not keen on this idea as they wanted to remain anonymous and feared possible repercussions from their local community. This was an important reminder of the need to work flexibly with young people and involve them in all stages of project planning.

**Contact**: Clare Jackson, Blackburn with Darwen Teenage Pregnancy Partnership
Clare.Jackson@bwdpct.nhs.uk
01254 267 000

## Developing information resources

There are many opportunities to turn the process of developing an information leaflet, logo, poster or video into a creative participation project for young people. Rather than consulting young people on how much they like a product created by adults, try to get young people involved in the whole process of developing a resource.

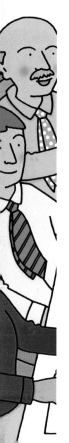

### Case study: Young people get resourceful

Young people have been involved in the planning and design of a range of resources as part of Wakefield's teenage pregnancy strategy, including a directory of local services and a series of posters. Most recently young people have been involved in the creation of a new teenage pregnancy and parenthood website. A questionnaire was distributed to more than 400 young people in a local school and Connexions centre to ask them what sort of information they would like to be included on the site. This included a competition for young people to decide what they thought the website should be called – the young people chose www.wakeyruready.co.uk

Young people from the school also spent time during their Personal, Social and Health Education (PSHE) lessons developing the more detailed content of the site, including questions and answers, case studies and story boards. The young people involved in writing the case studies have been accredited for their work and have achieved a Level 2 Open College Network Youth Training accreditation in sexual health.

The website was launched at an 'Inclusive Partnership' event where the young people helped to organise a workshop about the website for local professionals.

**Key learning**: Rather than arranging to meet young people straight after school, when they are often tired and hungry, it is a good idea to give them a break and meet up with them a bit later on once they have had a chance to recover from a busy school day.

**Contact**: Natalie Wain, Wakefield Teenage Pregnancy Partnership
Natalie.Wain@wwpct.nhs.uk
01924 213 051

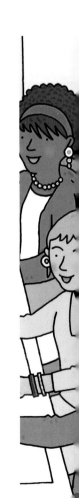

## Delivering services

One way to ensure that services are 'young-people-friendly' is to directly involve young people in certain aspects of service delivery. This can help make services more attractive and accessible to young people, and create significant opportunities for them to gain new skills.

### Case study: Sure Start Plus peer mentors

Sure Start Plus in Nottingham City recruited five peer mentors to provide additional support to the existing team of advisers and to offer information, support and advice to other pregnant teenagers and young

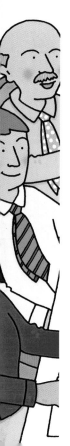

parents. Three young mums and two young dads were employed with support through the scheme to lead on this work and to complete Level 3 in mentoring as part of a National Vocational Qualification (NVQ).

Young people have responded well to the support they have received from the peer mentors. Their feedback suggests that they find the peer mentors more credible than some professionals from other agencies, who can sometimes ignore their needs or seem patronising. The peer mentors are dedicated to their work and want to see a positive difference to the lives of other young parents. The clear empathy and shared common experiences between the mentors and service users has added value to the adviser team and helped increased the capacity of the service.

**Key learning**: Despite the excellent outcomes of the work, a few difficulties were encountered. The mentoring scheme was offered short-term funding that led to a tight timescale. Sure Start Plus felt that the recruitment and induction of the mentors was rushed and, ideally, they would have liked to include service users on the interview panel for the mentors.

Staff would also have benefited from more time to develop a framework for the work in advance of the young people being recruited, so that effective support structures and systems of accountability were in already in place rather than evolving as the scheme progressed. With hindsight, staff also feel that it might have been beneficial to recruit slightly older young people, as some of the mentors still needed help to address their own support needs.

**Contact**: Judith Green, Nottingham City Sure Start Plus
Judith.green@nottinghamcity-pct.nhs.uk
0115 912 9287

### Case study: Peer educators distribute condoms

Young people have been trained as peer educators to distribute condoms to their peers in local high schools as part of Northumberland's 'c-card scheme'. This scheme was introduced in response to the need to develop a formal condom distribution scheme for young people in the area. The idea of involving peer educators in the scheme was introduced to increase the capacity of school nurses, to make the scheme as accessible as possible, and to provide the peer educators with opportunities to develop new skills.

The school nurses retain responsibility for the initial registration of young people to the c-card scheme and for the provision of basic education about sexual health issues, including condom demonstrations. The peer educators then distribute condoms when young people come back for more, and also provide informal advice and information. The school nurses provide the peer educators with comprehensive training before they start on the scheme. This consists of four evening sessions covering basic administration, safe use of condoms, condom clichés, confidentiality, and sex and the law.

The scheme has now been running for over three years. The informal approach of the peer educators has helped to optimise uptake of the scheme by young people. The peer educators themselves also benefit from valuable learning opportunities, and are rewarded for their achievements with certificates and annual c-card celebration events.

**Key learning**: It is vital to get the support of school headteachers and governors when developing opportunities for young people to get involved in peer education and condom distribution.

**Contact**: Jane Telfer, Northumberland Teenage Pregnancy Partnership
Jane.telfer@northumberlandcaretrust.nhs.uk
01670 819 049

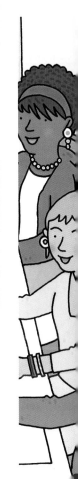

## Involving young people in staff training

Involving young people in staff training is a great way to bring a subject to life and enable adults to learn about young people's needs and perspectives from the experts. It also creates opportunities for young people to learn a range of skills required for delivering effective training, such as presentation and facilitation skills.

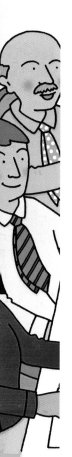

**Case study: Young mothers help the professionals**

Suffolk Teenage Pregnancy Partnership worked with its local Connexions, Sure Start and youth services to involve a group of young mothers in a project to help professionals increase their understanding of the needs of young mothers and improve their skills in communicating with young people.

An accredited training course was developed to enable the young mothers to develop their presentation and facilitation skills and identify key issues that they wanted professionals to take on board. Then they put their new skills to the test by presenting at a range of workshops and training events. They also created a range of fun training resources including a snakes and ladders game to illustrate the barriers facing young parents and the support they need to move forward.

The input from the young people has been very well received by professionals. Their feedback illustrates that the training helped to increase their understanding of the needs of young parents, and acted as a prompt for staff to review and develop their practice. The young mothers also gained new skills and confidence from their involvement in the project, and an increased ability to trust and communicate with professionals.

**Key learning**: It is vital to ensure that participation projects are firmly embedded within organisations so the work can be sustained when key individuals leave.

**Contact**: Sharon Singleton, Suffolk Teenage Pregnancy Partnership
Sharon.Singleton@connexionssuffolk.org.uk
01473 261 914

# Involving young people in staff recruitment

Without seeing people in action we can only guess at how well they are able to communicate with young people. Involving young people in the process of recruiting new staff is a great way to see these crucial skills in action and ensure that services are run by staff with the necessary motivation and skills to work effectively with young people. As well as involving young people in the actual interviews you may also want them to help with the process of writing the job description and shortlisting applications for interview (Michael and others 2002).

**Case study: Young people put interviewees in the hot seat**

A multi-agency team in Cumbria consisting of staff from Connexions and from teenage pregnancy and sexual health services involved young people in interviews for the recruitment of a young women's community health worker. Two young women were recruited to take part in the interviews through links with local voluntary youth organisations.

Prior to the interviews the young people received training to learn basic interview techniques, clarify their role and responsibilities, and plan what questions they wanted to ask. Following the interviews the young people took part in a full and frank discussion with the adults to agree on the successful candidate. They enjoyed their involvement in the interviews and gained new skills and confidence from the experience. Their involvement also created a relaxed atmosphere for the candidates and enabled them to demonstrate to the panel how they interact with young people and establish a rapport.

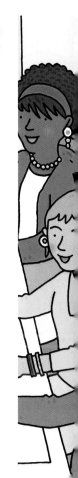

The benefits of involving the young people in making this decision have since been demonstrated by the success with which the post-holder effectively engages young women in work to promote their health and well-being. Evidence of these positive outcomes has also led to an increased commitment to involving young people in the interview process across services for children and young people in Cumbria.

**Key learning**: Interviews inevitably generate differences in opinion between both adults and young people, so it is important to agree in advance how a consensus will be reached on final decisions.

**Contact**: Christine Clark, Cumbria Teenage Pregnancy Partnership
Christine.clark@cumbriacc.gov.uk
01228 601 207

## Involving young people in policy and planning

There are many ways to directly involve young people in policy and planning to ensure that decisions are rooted in their needs and experiences. Rather than consulting young people on documents drafted by adults, consider how young people can be involved in the whole process of developing policies and plans.

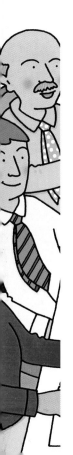

### Case study: Care leavers get animated about sex and relationships

Somerset Teenage Pregnancy Partnership worked with its leaving care project worker to involve care leavers in a consultation for a new sex and relationships policy to guide professional practice for young people in and leaving care.

The young people were encouraged to reflect on their own experiences of receiving advice and support about sex and relationships issues and their ideas for how this could be improved for other young people. They then worked with a participative arts worker to create a short animated film to communicate their views and recommendations. Their recommendations included the need for greater confidentiality about young people between social workers and foster carers, and a policy for young people written in a language they can relate to.

The film was shown at an event for senior service managers. The young people's recommendations were listened to with interest and a commitment was given to take them forward. Following their involvement in the project the young people were keen to get involved in future projects to improve the quality of support for their peers. The next step will be for the children's social care participation worker to involve looked-after children in the development of a young people's guide to sex and relationships.

**Key learning**: The young people were initially sceptical about anything happening or changing as a result of making the film. The event with senior service managers helped to counter this scepticism by giving young people a direct opportunity to learn how their work would lead to change.

**Contact**: Julie Husband, Somerset Teenage Pregnancy Partnership
Jhusband@connexions-somerset.org.uk
01823 320 309

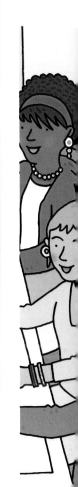

## Case study: Action planning 'away days'

Northumberland Teenage Pregnancy Partnership organises annual action planning 'away days' as one way to ensure that their local strategy is developed in direct response to the needs and experiences of young people. The away days represent an opportunity for practitioners to work in partnership with young people to reflect on progress from the previous year and look at what needs to happen in the next year. At least half of the participants at the away day are young people and they are recruited to represent a diversity of needs, including pregnant teenagers and young parents, users of local sexual health services, and pupils from a local pupil referral unit.

The away days start with icebreakers to create a relaxed atmosphere. Ground rules are then agreed in order to ensure a safe environment. This is followed by group work facilitated by staff with experience of working with young people. At the last event young people raised a number of issues including the need for a teen-specific sexual health magazine and improved debt advice for young parents. Both of these ideas have since been followed up with action and are included in the strategy.

Following the events, young people are given gift vouchers and letters of recognition. They are also sent copies of the draft strategy and are given the opportunity to feed back their comments and ideas. The events have helped to promote young people's participation in other work, as young people have gone on to speak at conferences and to facilitate workshops for professionals.

**Key learning**: The events have served to remind the team of the importance of getting young people's feedback on the events so that the format and focus evolve in a way that most effectively engages young people.

**Contact**: Judith Stonebridge, Northumberland Teenage Pregnancy Partnership
Judith.Stonebridge@northumberlandcaretrust.nhs.uk
01670 819 049

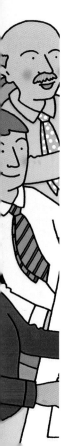

## Involving young people in advisory groups and boards

Involving young people in advisory groups or boards is a useful way of enabling young people to feed into decision-making processes and have a dialogue with adults on a long-term or ongoing basis. This can enable a more in-depth exploration and consideration of issues, including all the complexities and dilemmas. You might want to set up a group of young people who meet separately from adults and feed into key decision-making, or you might also want young people to directly attend meetings with adults where the decisions get made. Why not ask young people what they prefer (see Akpeki 2001).

## Case study: Young people get on board

Suffolk Teenage Pregnancy Partnership and Suffolk Connexions Partnership share a Partnership Board. They have established a Parallel Board for young people, to work alongside the adult Board and influence decision-making. Its members have been recruited to represent a cross-section of young people from across the county. This includes pupils from local schools and colleges, teenage parents, and young people not in education or training.

Two weeks before the Partnership Board meets, the Parallel Board holds meetings with the chief executive and the independent chair of the Partnership Board to discuss a shared agenda. Notes from these meetings are then discussed with the Partnership Board. Members of the Parallel Board meet in locality groups prior to the Parallel Board meetings to ensure that a wide range of opinions and ideas inform the discussion. The format of the meetings is informal, helping to create a safe space where young people feel relaxed and confident to voice their opinions openly and honestly.

The Parallel Board has provided a valuable forum for young people to discuss and inform issues that affect them. For example, young people in Suffolk have discussed the implications of the *Youth Matters* Green Paper and informed a bid to the DfES to pilot the 'Youth Opportunity Card', which encourages disadvantaged young people to participate in regular constructive activity. They have also helped to shape decisions about the local provision of sex and relationship education.

**Key learning**: It was initially planned that young people would attend the adult board meetings rather than meet separately. The change of plan evolved in response to the needs of young people, as they felt meeting separately would provide more scope for free and full discussions. This shows the importance of building plans around the needs of young people and empowering them to participate in a style and format that suits them best.

**Contact**: Pauline Henry, Connexions Suffolk
Pauline.Henry@connexionssuffolk.org.uk
01473 261 914

## Involving young people in conferences and events

Creating opportunities for young people to get involved in conferences and events can be an excellent way of enabling them to share findings from projects they have been involved in and communicate their views and experiences to influence local practitioners and policy-makers.

**Case study: Every Young Person Matters conference**

Nottingham City and Nottinghamshire County Teenage Pregnancy Partnerships worked together to involve young people in a conference on the five themes of the Every Child Matters programme. The event aimed to provide an opportunity for strategic leads, service commissioners and service managers to listen to the needs of local young people.

A diverse range of young people made presentations on each of the five themes to communicate their experiences of local services and make recommendations on how they could be improved. These included presentations by young parents and a short play by a group of care leavers to highlight the need for well-integrated services. A video of young people talking about their views and experiences of local services was also shown at the event. This was made to ensure that less confident young people also had opportunities to have their voices heard by local decision-makers.

Feedback from the event was very positive and reflected a high level of commitment to act upon young people's views in the future design and delivery of services. A report was produced to feed this information back to the young people who took part and demonstrate that their input had made a positive difference.

**Key learning**: The success of the event highlighted the importance of inviting delegates who are in a position to affect change, and who may not otherwise have regular opportunities to communicate directly with young people.

**Contact**: Sue Jablonskas, Nottinghamshire County Teenage Pregnancy Partnership

Sue.Jablonskas@nottscc.gov.uk
0115 915 7028

Irene Kakoullis, Nottingham City Teenage Pregnancy Partnership
Irene.Kakoullis@nottinghamcity.gov.uk
01623 627 322

## Involving young people in the media

There is great potential for young people to get involved in local and
national media to raise awareness of issues related to sexual health and
teenage pregnancy. Young people often find messages about sex and
relationships more credible when their peers communicate them. There are
a wide range of media activities in which young people can get involved,
including writing articles for newspapers and magazines, or taking part in
radio or television programmes. Some TPPs have also provided young
people with training to help them gain the confidence and skills to talk
about teenage pregnancy issues in the local and national media.

**Case study: Spreading the message via the media**

Enfield and Haringey Teenage Pregnancy Team have involved young people
in a range of projects to communicate key messages about sex and
relationships in the local media. Young people have composed songs about
safe sex and produced radio adverts to publicise local sexual health
services, which have been played on local community radio stations. They
have also produced a short TV advert that has been shown on TV screens in
local buses and shopping centres.

A diverse group of young people were recruited from local agencies
including the Youth Offending Team, Connexions, 4YP services, and
services for care leavers and asylum-seekers. A group of young mothers
have also produced a 10-minute film for their peers, which includes top
tips and advice about being a new mum.

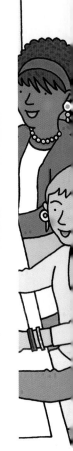

Young people also attend a media working group that has been established to inform the development of local media work.

**Key learning**: Remember that working with groups of energetic young people can be demanding – having two or more facilitators works well to keep the momentum going and capture young people's interest and enthusiasm.

**Contact**: Joan Badcock, Enfield and Haringey Teenage Pregnancy Partnership
joan.badcock@haringey.gov.uk
020 8489 2952

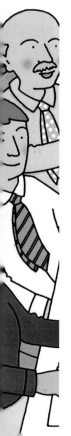

# 4 Creating the conditions for effective participation

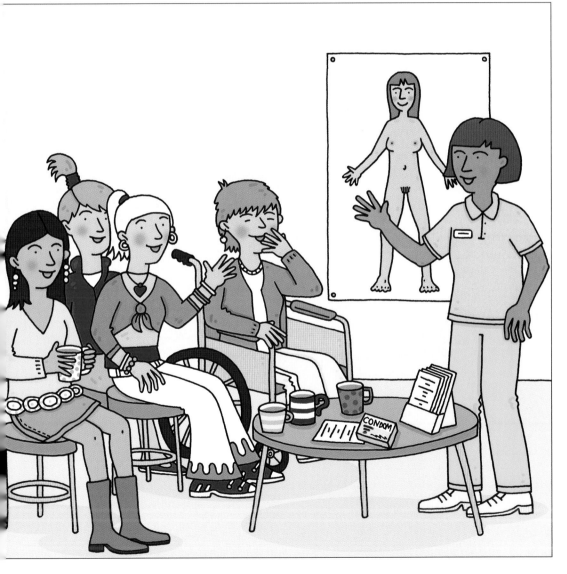

**It feels good to express myself and say what I think about things.**

**(young person)**

# 4 Creating the conditions for effective participation

This section provides an outline of ways organisations can increase opportunities for young people to actively participate in their work. It is of particular relevance to managers, as they have an important role in building capacity for young people to get involved in decision-making.

## Your starting point

It is important to take stock of how young people are currently involved in your work and to establish this as a starting point for making future plans. Reflecting on what you have done in the past can help you to identify what went well, what could have been different, and what else is needed in the future. Once you have established your starting point you will be in a good position to identify the best way to build on the work and strengthen the experience and confidence of your team.

## Support from the top

For young people to be effectively involved in the work of an organisation, staff at all levels need to be prepared to do things differently. Support for the concept of young people's participation is needed at the very highest organisational level. Leaders and managers of organisations have an important role in building a culture of participation within which staff are supported and encouraged to involve young people in their work. They

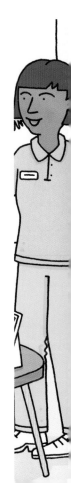

also need to make sure that resources and time are set aside for participation work to take place; young people's views are acted upon; and participation is integrated into work right across the organisation.

**A lesson learned...**

> ...a group of young people we were working with at the Youth Service wanted to see more leisure facilities for young people in their local area, so we encouraged them to write letters to their local Councillor to express their views and ask whether they could help. We wanted the young people to feel empowered but they were crestfallen when they received their reply as the letter was fairly dismissive and pointed out their spelling mistakes. The experience highlighted the need to work with partners to develop a shared understanding of participation, and the importance of a shared commitment from the top-down. (practitioner)

## Training and support for staff

Participation needs to be integral to the role of all staff working to support young people. Training can be a useful way to enable staff to gain a shared understanding of participation and develop their practice. Many of the key national organisations that focus on young people's participation can provide training. Further information on available training resources and providers can be found in References and further information (page 65). You may also find local agencies that can provide training at a low cost.

Managers can also support ongoing learning and reflection by encouraging staff to discuss participation during supervision and to make links with local or national participation initiatives. Some organisations have benefited from creating dedicated posts to help staff develop their skills and confidence in involving young people.

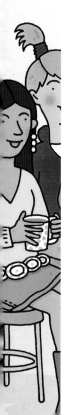

**Case study: Helping staff to involve young people**

Nottingham City Teenage Pregnancy Partnership established a participation worker post to help consolidate young people's involvement in local work to prevent teenage pregnancy and support young parents. Alongside direct work with young people on a range of participation projects, the role also involves assisting practitioners from other agencies to effectively involve young people in their work. To achieve this the participation worker has developed and delivered a training programme for staff working in the teenage pregnancy field. The training covers participation theory and practical advice on how to involve young people in the design and delivery of services. The training has adopted the 'Ready Steady Change' training model developed by the Children's Rights Alliance.

Training for key workers has helped to embed participation within local services and has led to changing attitudes to working effectively with young people. Some practitioners are concerned about not having the skills to actively involve young people, and the training has been useful in increasing their confidence in this area of work.

**Key learning**: Outcomes from the training highlight the importance of providing practitioners with tools to help them to apply their learning to their work.

**Contact**: Irene Kakoullis, Nottingham City Teenage Pregnancy Partnership
Irene.Kakoullis@nottinghamcity.gov.uk
0115 969 1177

## Financial considerations

Access to sufficient financial resources is vital if you want to provide fun and creative opportunities for young people to get involved in the work of your organisation. As well as the costs entailed in carrying out the participation work, it often costs money to act on the suggestions that young people make. If you have lots of ideas but limited resources it can

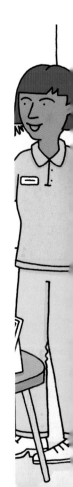

be a good idea to pool budgets with partner organisations and investigate the possibility of getting financial help from local and national grant-giving bodies.

## Working together

Working in partnership will help to maximise opportunities for young people to participate in decision-making processes. By working together we can help to build a shared approach to participation and provide the consistent and integrated services needed to promote young people's health and well-being.

> You need to be able to call on other agencies – it's hard to keep
> the momentum going on your own.
> (practitioner)

Children's Trusts (to be rolled out from April 2006) will be well positioned to lead on work to develop shared approaches to participation, such as setting up networks and forums to enhance existing practice. This could also involve developing and implementing participation standards, including those devised by national voluntary organisations (see Wade and Badham 2003 and Northwest Children's Taskforce 2002). For example, organisations in a given area may agree to include participatory working practices in the job description for all posts involving work with children and young people.

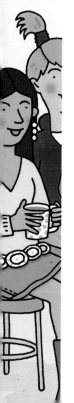

### Case study: Young 'change agents' shape Children's Trust

Young people's participation has been given a high priority in the development of Leicester Federation, which is a pathfinder Children's Trust. The Federation is a partnership consisting of all the agencies working with children and young people in Leicester. It has taken a number of steps to ensure that children and young people are actively involved in decisions about the design and delivery of local service provision. A participation sub-group has been established to develop and support implementation of a participation strategy in local agencies including the Teenage Pregnancy Partnership, Social Care and Health, Lifelong Learning and the Children's Fund. The objectives of the strategy are to:

- establish shared values within and across partner agencies
- secure agreed standards within and across partner agencies
- ensure coordination and coherence across partner agencies
- ensure monitoring and review across partner agencies.

Agencies are working to adopt the National Youth Agency's 'Hear By Right' participation standards within all Federation partner organisations. The sub-group supports this process by providing opportunities for agencies to network and share learning.

Young people are also directly involved in the design and implementation of the participation strategy. Fifteen young people aged between 8 and 18 years have been recruited as local 'change agents' to feed into decision-making across the Federation. They were recruited via local agencies to represent a diverse range of young people, including looked after children, those excluded from school, and black and minority ethnic communities. The group, who have called themselves TALK (Think About Leicester's Kids) have so far concentrated on outlining key proposals under the seven standards of 'Hear By Right'. TALK's proposals have been included as underlying organisational principles in the development of Leicester's first statutory single Children and Young People's Plan. They have also informed strategic actions within the plan, including a proposal to increase peer education, support and mentoring schemes in all local agencies.

**Key learning**: When setting up a group similar to TALK it is important to find dedicated resources and not rely on partner agencies giving their time voluntarily in the long term, as competing commitments can threaten the sustainability of the work. It is also important to be prepared for progress to be slow, and ensure that young people and senior members of staff have a clear understanding of their respective roles from the outset. Another key lesson has been that partner agencies need to be clear about

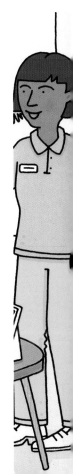

the role of the group. It is important that TALK and similar groups are not seen as representative of all children and young people and as a substitute for the participation work that should be undertaken by all agencies.

**Contact**: Mary-Ann Rickwood, Leicester Federation of Children's Services
Mary-Ann.Rickwood@leicester.gov.uk
0116 252 8190

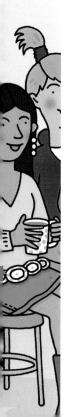

### Case study: Multi-agency participation group in Wakefield

Wakefield Children and Young People's Strategic Partnership has established a multi-agency sub-group to celebrate and promote participative practice among partner organisations that work with children and young people. The Involving Children and Young People Group currently involves representatives from a wide breadth of organisations including social services, the Young People's Service, the Local Education Authority, Connexions, the Teenage Pregnancy Service and Wakefield Children's Fund. Alongside this core 'executive group' a broader stakeholder group has also been established to draw in representation from a wider network of local agencies working with children and young people. The stakeholder group comes together periodically to learn about the work of the 'executive group' and act as a network through which to identify, develop and promote best practice.

The Involving Children and Young People Group has been operational since October 2004, in which time it has successfully written a participation strategy for Wakefield, 'Engaging with our Futures', which has been endorsed by the Wakefield Children and Young People's Strategic Partnership. The strategy sets ambitious targets, seeking not only to strengthen existing good practice, but to promote culture change where necessary so that the participation of children and young people in service design, delivery and review becomes the accepted norm among all agencies that have an impact on the lives of children and young people.

The strategy also sets out to address particular issues in an effort to establish shared best practice. These issues include responding to children and young people's complaints and compliments, their involvement in recruitment, and how children and young people are rewarded for their participation. The group is also ensuring that young people's views are sought throughout the deployment of the strategy by engaging with new and existing networks of children and young people.

**Key learning**: Competing priorities and busy workloads can make it difficult to gain the commitment of partner agencies. To counter this it is important to be clear with partner agencies from the outset about how their involvement will add value to their own work.

**Contact**: Natalie Wain, Wakefield Teenage Pregnancy Partnership
Natalie.Wain@wwpct.nhs.uk
01924 213 05

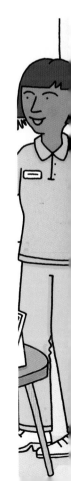

# 5 Directory of partners in participation

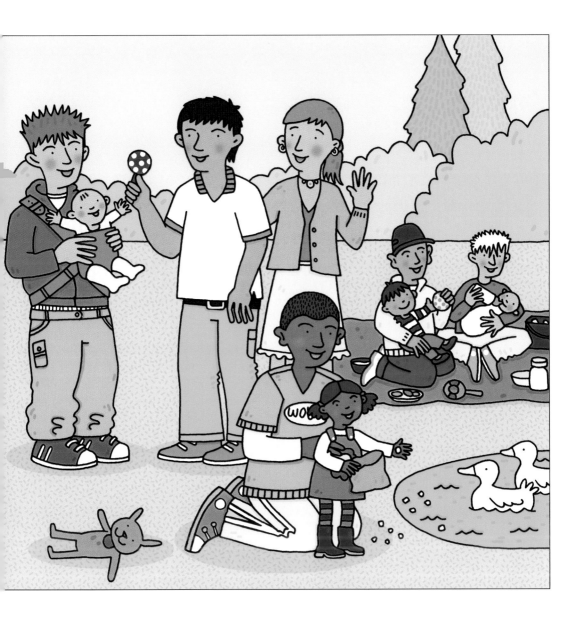

**Our opinions are important and can help services to change.**

**(young person)**

# 5 Directory of partners in participation

This section provides an overview of some of the key agencies that have a role in creating opportunities for young people to participate in decision-making at a local level. You may want to contact some of these agencies to explore opportunities for joint work or potential funding opportunities.

## Children's Fund

Children and young people's participation is one of the three underlying principles of the Children's Fund programme. For information on the 35 national pathfinders see
**www.everychildmatters.gov.uk/strategy/childrensfund**

## Children's Trusts

Most top-tier local authorities in England will have a Children's Trust by April 2006. The effective involvement of children, young people and their families or carers is crucial to the development and running of all Children's Trusts. Contact your local authority for details on what is happening in your local area.

## Connexions

Listening to young people and taking account of their views is central to the ethos of Connexions. For details of your local Connexions Partnership go to **www.connexions.gov.uk**

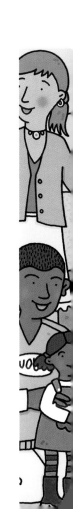

### Contraceptive and sexual health services (CASH)

Empowering and involving people who use services is crucial to the implementation of the National Strategy for Sexual Health and HIV. Contact your local primary care trust for information on local CASH services.

### Crime and disorder reduction partnerships/community safety partnerships

Guidance for local crime and disorder reduction partnerships emphasises the importance of involving children and young people in the development of local strategies. Further information on local partnerships can be found at **www.crimereduction.gov.uk**

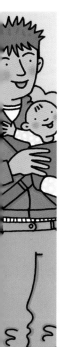

### Drug Action Teams (DATs)

A central aim of the government's drug strategy is to ensure provision is built around the needs of vulnerable children and young people. Young people's involvement is essential to the successful design and delivery of local DAT plans regarding young people's substance misuse. A list of DATs can be found at **www.drugs.gov.uk/dat/directory**

### General practice

The general practice (GP) contract emphasises the need to involve patients fully in treatment decisions and to seek their feedback to improve the quality of service provision. For information on GP surgeries in your area see **www.nhs.uk/england/doctors**

### Healthy Care

Healthy Care provides support and guidance to local healthy care partnerships to develop a programme of work to promote the participation and health and well-being of looked after children and young people. Further information on local partnerships is available at **www.ncb.org.uk/healthycare**

## Healthy Schools

At a local level, healthy schools programmes provide support to schools in becoming healthier places for staff and pupils to work and learn, based on the key principle of young people's active participation. For details of healthy schools programmes in your area contact your primary care trust and local education authority, or go to **www.wiredforhealth.gov.uk**

## Maternity services for young parents

Standard 11 of the National Service Framework (NSF) for Child Health and Maternity Services emphasises the need for maternity services to ensure that parents (including teenage parents) are involved in the planning and evaluation of services and are supported to make informed choices about their care. Your local primary care trust (PCT) will be able to provide you with information on maternity services in your area. For details of your local PCT go to **www.nhs.uk/england/authoritiestrusts/pct**

## Pharmacies

Standard 10 of the NSF states that the expertise of pharmacists should be used in supporting wider health promotion strategies for children and young people. This entails involving young people to ensure services are designed around their needs. For details of pharmacies in your local area contact your PCT or go to **www.nhs.uk/england/pharmacies**

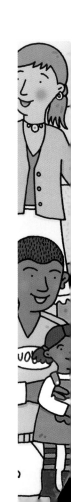

## Primary care trusts, strategic health authorities and NHS trusts

Patient and public involvement forums (PPI forums) exist in NHS trusts and PCTs to improve the quality of NHS services by bringing to trusts and PCTs the views and experiences of patients, their carers and families. There is an expectation that young people are involved in PPI forums and initiatives at a local level. Contact your PCT for information on PPI initiatives in your area. For details of your local PCT go to **www.nhs.uk/england/authoritiestrusts/pct**

## Schools and colleges

The importance of pupil participation in decision-making within schools and colleges is enshrined in policy and fundamental to delivery of the Citizenship agenda. Many schools have established school councils, which can be a valuable forum for involving young people in wider decisions about their local community. Contact your LEA for more information. For details of your LEA go to **www.dfes.gov.uk/localauthorities**

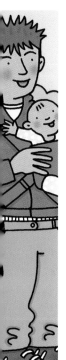

## Secure settings

Local authority secure children's homes, secure training centres and young offender institutions work to ensure that young people have an opportunity to participate in decision-making within custody and the wider community. Contact details for secure facilities can be found on the Youth Justice Board website at **www.youth-justice-board.gov.uk**

## Social services

Local authorities with social services responsibilities have the power to scrutinise health services as part of their role in reducing health inequalities. Guidance emphasises the importance of involving children and young people in the process of scrutinising services that affect them.

## Substance misuse services

National Treatment Agency guidance states that the involvement of young people in decisions about their treatment, and operational planning is fundamental to effective young people's substance misuse treatment services. Contact your local Drug Action Team for details of local services.

## Supported housing

The Supporting People initiative requires providers of supported housing to place a strong emphasis on user participation and to involve service users in decisions made about the design and delivery of services. Contact your local council housing department for a list of local supported housing services for young people, including teenage parents.

## Sure Start Children's Centres

Parental involvement is one of the key principles of Sure Start. Contact details for local programmes can be found on the Sure Start website at **www.surestart.gov.uk**

## Teenage Pregnancy Partnerships

Teenage Pregnancy Partnerships have a responsibility to ensure that young people participate in the design and delivery of local strategies to reduce teenage pregnancy and support young parents. Contact details for your local teenage pregnancy coordinator can be found on the Teenage Pregnancy Unit website at **www.dfes.gov.uk/teenagepregnancy**

## Youth and community services

Participation has long been central to the aim and ethos of the youth service. In any local area there is likely to be a range of statutory and voluntary projects working to empower young people and provide

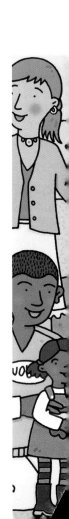

opportunities for them to get actively involved in their local community. Contact your local council to find out about youth projects and services in your local area.

## Youth Offending Teams

Youth Offending Teams work to ensure that the views and experiences of young people inform their annual youth justice plans. Contact details for all Youth Offending Teams can be found on the Youth Justice Board website at **www.youth-justice-board.gov.uk**

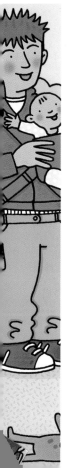

# 6 References and further information

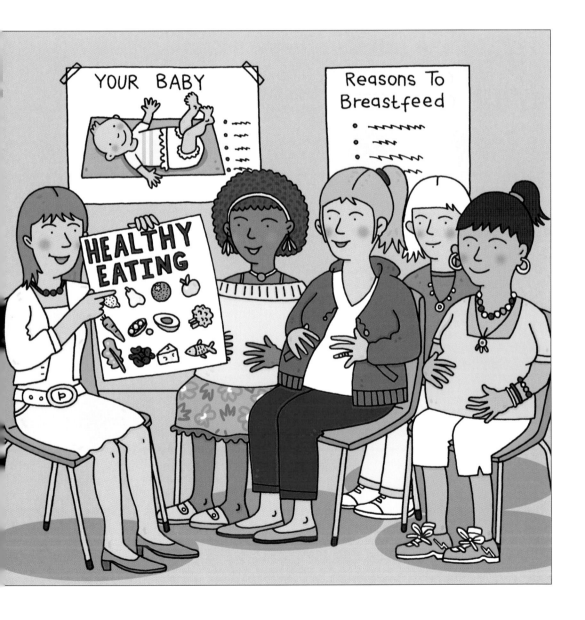

Thank you for listening to me and hearing my point of view.

(young person)

# 6 References and further information

## References

Akpeki, T (2001) *Guide to Board Development: Involving young people.* London: National Children's Bureau.

Blake, S and Frances, G (2004) *Giving Pupils a Voice: Promoting participation in healthy schools.* London: Department for Education and Skills and National Children's Bureau.

Brody, R (1998) *Getting Through: Young people and communication.* Brighton: Trust for the Study of Adolescence.

Department for Education and Skills (2004) *Every Child Matters: Change for Children.* Norwich: The Stationery Office.

Department of Health (2004a) *National Service Framework for children, young people and maternity services.* London: The Stationery Office.

Department of Health (2004b) *Choosing Health: Making healthy choices easier.* London: The Stationery Office.

Fajerman and others (2000) *Children As Partners In Planning: A training resource to support consultation with children.* London: Save the Children.

Hart, R (1997) *Children's Participation: The theory and practice of involving young citizens in community development and environmental care.* New York: UNICEF.

Hartley-Brewer, E (2002) *Stepping Forward – working together through peer support.* London: National Children's Bureau.

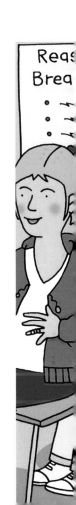

Jones, D (2003) *Communicating with Vulnerable Children: A guide for practitioners.* London: Gaskell.

Kirby, P (1999) *Involving Young Researchers: How to enable young people to design and conduct research.* London: Save the Children and Joseph Rowntree Foundation.

Kirby, P and others (2003) *Building a Culture of Participation: Involving children and young people in policy, service planning, delivery and evaluation.* London: Department for Education and Skills.

Kirkbride, L (1999) *I'll Go First: The planning and review toolkit for use with children with disabilities.* London: The Children's Society.

McCarthy, J (2004) *Enacting Participatory Development: Theatre-based techniques.* Trowbridge: Earthscan.

McGowan, M (2002) *Young People and Peer Support – how to set up a peer support programme.* Brighton: Trust for the Study of Adolescence.

Michael, E and others (2002) *Involving Young People In the Recruitment of Staff, Volunteers and Mentors.* London: National Children's Bureau.

Morris, J (1998) *Don't Leave Us Out – involving disabled children and young people with communication impairments.* York: Joseph Rowntree Foundation.

Northwest Children's Taskforce (2002) *Taking Part Toolkit: Promoting the 'real' participation of children and young people.* Barkingside, Essex: Barnardo's.

Shepherd, C and Treseder, P (2002) *Participation: Spice it up!* Swansea: Dynamix and Save the Children.

Wade, H and Badham, B (2003) *Hear By Right: Standards for the active involvement of children and young people.* Leicester: National Youth Agency.

Willow, C (2002) *Participation in Practice: Children and young people as partners in change.* London: The Children's Society.

Worall, S (2000) *Young People As Researchers: A learning resource pack.* London: Save the Children.

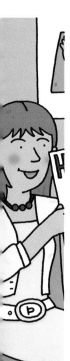

## Other useful publications

Children and Young People's Unit (2002) *Learning to Listen: Core principles for the involvement of children and young people*. London: Department for Education and Skills.

Children's Society (2002) *Young People's Charter of Participation*. London: The Children's Society.

Children's Rights Officers and Advocates (2000) *Total Respect!*. London: Department of Health.

Cutler, D (2002) *Taking the Initiative: Promoting young people's involvement in public decision-making in the UK*. London: Carnegie United Kingdom Trust.

Lightfoot, J and Sloper, P (2002) *Having a Say in Health: Guidelines for involving young patients in health service development*. York: University of York.

McNeish, D and Turner, C (2001) *A Guide to Involving Young People in Teenage Pregnancy Work*. London: Teenage Pregnancy Unit.

Treseder, P (1997) *Empowering Children and Young People*. London: Save the Children.

White, P (2001) *Local and Vocal: Promoting young people's involvement in local decision-making; an overview and planning guide*. London: Save the Children and National Youth Agency.

## Useful websites and organisations

Barnardo's
www.barnardos.org.uk
Barnardo's works with vulnerable children and young people in the UK and produces a range of resources for professionals. The 'Committed to Rights' section of the website gives information, examples and practical tools to help practitioners working in the criminal justice system make their work as participatory as possible: www.barnardos.co.uk/committedtorights

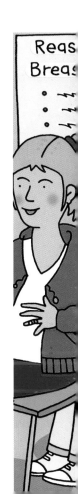

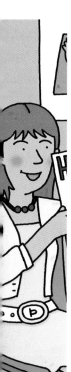

### British Youth Council (BYC)
www.byc.org.uk

BYC represents and involves a unique coalition of young people through their participation as individuals or through their youth organisations. BYC brings young people together to agree on issues of common concern and encourage them to bring about change through taking collective action.

### Carnegie Young People Initiative (CYPI)
www.carnegieuktrust.org.uk/cypi/home

Children's and young people's participation is the sole focus of CYPI, which specialises in research, new ideas, and piloting innovative projects. CYPI works to support not only children and young people, but practitioners and organisations seeking to change the way they work.

### Children's Rights Alliance for England (CRAE)
www.crae.org.uk

CRAE is a coalition of over 275 voluntary and statutory organisations committed to the fullest implementation of the UN Convention on the Rights of the Child. On the 'Ready Steady Change' section of the website you will find training, tools and an online library of resources to put children's and young people's wishes, feelings and ideas at the centre of public services.

### Citizenship Foundation
www.citizenshipfoundation.org.uk

The Citizenship Foundation aims to empower individuals to engage in the wider community through education about the law, democracy and society.

### National Children's Bureau (NCB)
www.ncb.org.uk

NCB promotes the voices, interests and well-being of all children and young people across every aspect of their lives. As an umbrella body for the children's sector in England and Northern Ireland, NCB provides essential information on policy, research and best practice for our members and other partners.

National Youth Agency (NYA)

www.nya.org.uk

The NYA supports those involved in young people's personal and social development and works to enable all young people to fulfil their potential within a just society. The 'Hear by Right' section of the website provides a tried and tested standards framework for organisations to assess and improve practice and policy on the active involvement of children and young people: www.nya.org.uk/hearbyright

Office of the Children's Commissioner

www.childrenscommissioner.org.uk

The Office of the Children's Commissioner is a non-departmental government body that has the general function of promoting awareness of the views and interests of children in England. The Children's Commissioner provides an independent, national voice for all children and young people, especially the disadvantaged and the vulnerable.

Participation Works

www.participationworks.org.uk

Participation Works is an online gateway to the world of children's and young people's participation. On the site you can access policy, practice, networks and information from across the UK. You can also share resources, learn about children's rights, search the knowledge hub or find out about innovative practice and new ideas.

Save the Children

www.savethechildren.org.uk

Save the Children has campaigned for the rights of children for over 80 years. The organisation's work in the UK aims to bring about long-term change for some of the most vulnerable children across the country: those growing up in poverty; those missing out on quality education; and those who have come to England to seek refuge and asylum.

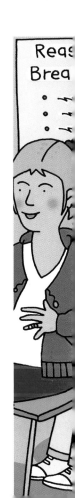

UK Youth Parliament (UKYP)

www.ukyouthparliament.org.uk

UKYP aims to give the young people of the UK between the ages of 11 and 18 a voice, which will be heard and listened to by local and national government, providers of services for young people and other agencies that have an interest in the views and needs of young people.

Young NCB

www.youngncb.org.uk

Young NCB is a free membership network run by NCB, open to all children and young people. As Young NCB members, young people can be actively involved in issues that affect and interest them, such as safety, perceptions of young people, sex and relationships education, bullying and drugs.

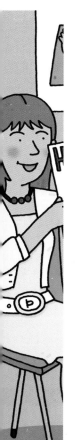